alive **Natural Health Guides 4**

Rhody L

Liver Cleansing
Handbook

How to keep
your liver happy

- **Eliminate toxins**
- **Rejuvenate your liver**
- **Overcome tiredness**
- **Energize your life**

alive
BOOKS
Vancouver
Canada

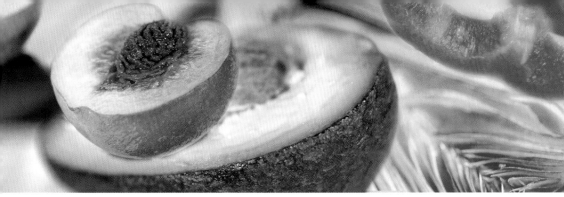

c o n t e n t s

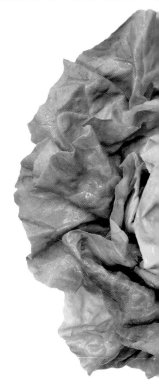

All About Liver Cleansing

Recipes

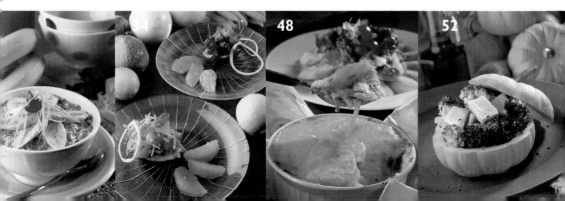

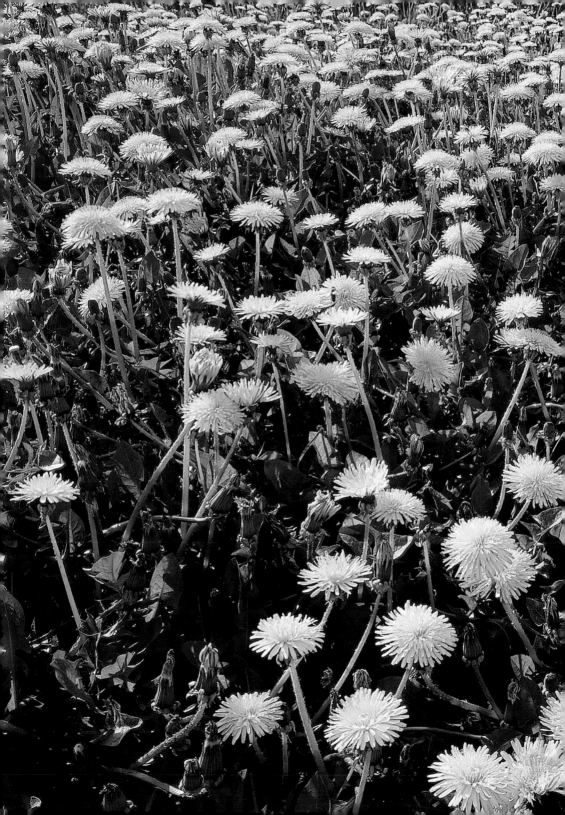

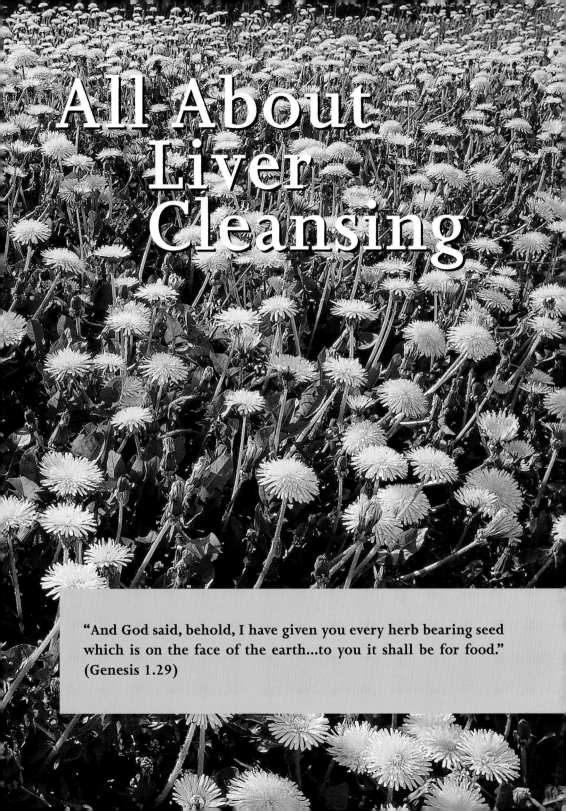

All About Liver Cleansing

"And God said, behold, I have given you every herb bearing seed which is on the face of the earth...to you it shall be for food." (Genesis 1.29)

The liver delivers all the necessary nutrients to cells, muscle and brain tissue, organs, glands, hair, nails–all the parts that make up "you."

Every organ, gland, muscle and tissue of the body functions together to make a harmonious and homogeneous whole, and the liver perhaps plays the most important role. Indeed, "liver" comes from the old English word for "life." Keeping your liver happy is essential to your life, so it's truly worthwhile to find out how to treat what the Chinese call "the father of all organs." Perhaps we should adopt the common Russian greeting, "How's your liver today?"

You're the only one responsible for choosing what you put into your body. Liver toxins can be found in the food you've been brought up on and that you love best!

You may be taking treatment for a number of health problems–constipation, allergies, high cholesterol, irritable bowel, high blood sugar, asthma, skin rashes–not knowing that the real problem stems from your liver. This large and very important detoxifying organ is clogged, sluggish, ailing, unhappy–in short, dysfunctional. And it's all the result of poor diet and lifestyle.

The good news is that the liver is very forgiving. Optimum liver function can be restored and even a damaged liver can be regenerated. It's all a matter of knowing what to do and what not to do. The purpose of this book is to motivate you to consider your liver and adopt a diet protocol that will allow your liver to detoxify daily. If you assist your liver to do its job well, you will function better on all cylinders, mentally, emotionally and physically.

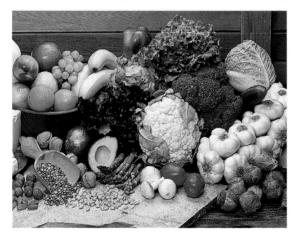

A Toxic World . . .

The liver works as part of a team in your body, and its job is to detoxify. The need to detoxify is more important than ever before because we live in a toxic environment, largely as a result of "advances" from the industrial revolution–agricultural chemicals used in farming, chemical food additives, pharmaceutical drugs, chlorination and fluoridation of water, car exhaust and indoor pollutants from chemical cleaners, paint, carpets and furniture. These substances all contribute to the general toxicity with which the body must cope.

But the greatest assault on the body and the liver is from modern food. Denatured, processed and chemicalized foods are unique to this century and cause greater stress on the liver than your ancestors experienced. Your liver must work constantly to eliminate these toxins through the lungs, skin, kidneys and bowels so that they do not get into the bloodstream. An overload of toxins means all organs are overloaded too, and each must do more than it can adequately handle. So, we get symptoms. Doctors call these symptoms "disease." Unfortunately, they usually treat the symptoms and never investigate the cause.

The most prevalent, and therefore the most insidious, of these toxins are trans-fatty acids from hydrogenated oils, which are in almost every processed or packaged food item in the supermarket. Hydrogenated oils are even found in some items in your health food store, and altogether now constitute upwards of forty-seven percent of the current dietary fat intake. These oils, artificially hardened by metal and hydrogen gas, produce fatty acid trans-isomers that are not natural to the human body. They're foreign, and your body does not know what to do with them. Adding processed, hydrogenated, manmade fats to your diet actually puts you in greater danger of heart disease, breast cancer and diabetes than if you consume animal fats.

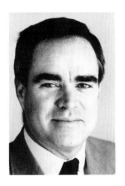

"The liver was not designed to deal with the pollutants that have become part of modern life in the past 100 years." – Guide to Natural Healing, Julian Whitaker, MD

7

The Body's Pathways of Detoxification

You have only one liver and you must keep it functioning properly for your body to detoxify. Since it's only the liver that can purify the bloodstream, you should keep your liver happy, regularly cleansing it by eating a daily regimen of specific foods and nutrients. Toxins are then easily excreted via prescribed pathways, through the gallbladder to bile to the bowels, and through the kidneys to the bladder.

Through these pathways, you eliminate micro-organisms (parasites), insecticides, food additives, fake fats, pharmaceutical drugs, alcohol and other toxins.

When these pathways are clogged or overloaded toxins must then be eliminated through the skin, resulting in eczema, acne rosacea, itchy skin, brownish skin blemishes, red, flushed face and skin rashes.

There's another problem. Even if you meticulously read labels you won't find trans-fatty acids listed as contents on the package. Manufacturers are not legally required to give you this information. In fact, the Canadian Health Protection Branch has ruled that "it is not in consumer interest" for you to know.

So if you have listened to the current hype to reduce fat intake, and eat "no-fat," "low-fat" and "fat-free" products, you may be ingesting less animal fat that you did ten years ago but the percentage of bad fat in your diet is still the same.

Now on the market are products like Olestra™, which is a fake fat that is designed to go right through your digestive system without being digested. This fake fat has been reported to cause severe intestinal cramps and other side effects. Your liver is severely compromised when it's asked to dispose of such toxins.

What is required is a new eating pattern and a liver-cleansing diet, one that will enable all the assisting organs—pancreas, kidneys, intestines, bowels—to function optimally. In such a case your liver never becomes blocked with toxic waste. And if your liver is handling natural fats, both vegetable and animal, manufacturing optimum amounts of cholesterol, and assisting in the production of bile, you'll be grooving! I guarantee it.

Bile Balance . . . .

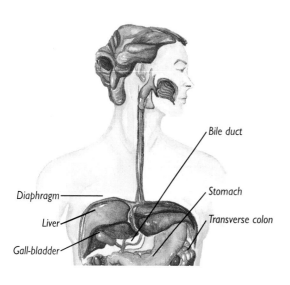

Diaphragm

Liver

Gall-bladder

Bile duct

Stomach

Transverse colon

Bile is essential. Bile is a bitter yellow-green fluid that is produced by the liver and stored in the gallbladder, where it is released as needed for digestion. Bile breaks down fat into small globules and assists in absorbing oils, fats and fat-soluble vitamins (A, D, E and K). It also helps to convert beta-carotene into vitamin A and frees the small intestine of potentially harmful micro-organisms. And it promotes peristalsis (movement) in the bowels to keep the feces moving along the digestive tract and out of the body as waste, thus preventing constipation–the bane of Western civilization.

Barring overindulgence, the normal digestive process once worked for humans as it should, and the liver was able to produce the bile necessary for digestion and elimination, keeping all the other pathways clear.

As we entered the revolution of modern machinery and technological innovations human health began to decline. Food became something other than the compounds the body understands and is able to metabolize. The liver suddenly had a huge job to do. It did not recognize the new altered foods, so it treated them as toxins and set about eliminating them from the body as best it could. When there were too many to remove through the normal digestive process, the liver tried to push them out through the skin. When the liver became overloaded and tired, the toxins stayed in the body, artificially hardened fats and other poisons circulated in the blood and the result is degeneration and disease.

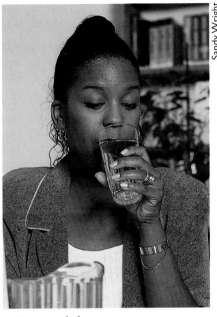

Drinking eight glasses of water a day is essential for a happy liver.

Your Liver or Your Life . . . .

The liver is designed to operate with clocklike precision. At about two o'clock in the morning it begins to sort out the nutrients received from the last meal. If that meal has been light and not eaten too late in the day your liver can easily manage, sending sufficient bile to the gallbladder for the next stage of digestion. If you eat a heavy meal and eat too late, your liver works overtime–until about eight in the morning, or later–but with no extra pay! That sluggish liver will keep you between the covers in the morning, not wanting to get up. You'll be grumpy and complain that you're not a "morning person." In reality you're "liverish." Your liver has not been able to get rid of its toxic load. So you start the day with a cup of coffee to get a jump start, but the caffeine compromises the liver even more. You may then have a bagel and cream cheese for breakfast, more coffee mid-morning and French fries with your pizza for lunch!

The liver's response to the caffeine, sugar and hydrogenated fats is frantic! More toxic overload! And if your regular diet also includes packaged cookies, crackers, chips, dips, breads and spreads full of trans-fatty acids and chemical additives, your liver will eventually give up.

Liver Distress Signals . . . .

When you feel fatigued, listless, at odds with the world, that's your liver talking. Even young people can have a clogged and toxin-loaded liver, which does not bode well for their future health. Young people on a diet of fast and processed foods can expect an ongoing series of symptoms that medical doctors are trained to treat with prescription drugs (thereby adding to the body's toxicity) with no knowledge or understanding of the underlying cause–a miserable liver!

Some of the signals of liver distress include:	
• high blood pressure	• eczema, acne rosacea, pimples
• elevated cholesterol	• chronic fatigue syndrome
• weight gain	• brownish spots on the skin
• pot belly	(liver spots)
• cellulite	• hot flashes
• indigestion	• compromised pancreas
• abdominal bloating	• depression
• irritable bowel syndrome	• irritability

The list goes on.

Most North Americans don't get the message. They treat the symptoms with over-the-counter or prescription drugs, and carry on with their liver-destroying lifestyles.

If you've decided to change all that, this book will help you to be your own doctor and achieve better health.

Easing the Digestion Process . . . .

Proper digestion starts with knowing what you should eat. Perhaps the answers appear obvious, but maybe you have some misconceptions about what constitutes a "healthy" diet.

First, are you aware that most of the packaged food in your supermarket–those that fill most shoppers' grocery carts–contain chemical additives and preservatives? The list is as long as your arm and includes arsenic, hydroxide of ammonia, ascetic anhydride, sodium hypochlorite, calcium aluminum silicate and magnesium stearate, to name a few. Food colors are made up of chemical dyes with unpronounceable names that neither the consumer nor the body understands. Check out books like *Hard to Swallow: The Truth About Food Additives* (alive books, 1999), that tell you about the toxins manufacturers put in your food.

We should be eating fresh, whole fruit and vegetables, cooked as lightly as possible; cooked grains and legumes; fresh, raw nuts and seeds; whole-grain bread and cereal without chemical additives. The kind of food your ancestors ate.

Digestion begins in the mouth, and food should be well salivated through chewing. And though daily intake of water is essential (eight glasses a day), do not drink water with meals. Drink water two hours after a meal or half an hour before meals as a general rule. Consuming liquids with meals dilutes digestive juices and important hydrochloric acid. You need these stomach juices and acids to digest food easily and quickly, to destroy any bacteria that may be in the food you eat and to facilitate rapid bowel function. With sufficient hydrochloric acid in the stomach, vitamins and minerals are properly utilized. Without enough of the acid, food putrefies in the stomach, thereby causing gas, bloating and discomfort. Your liver will be stymied and won't be able to do its job.

Older people are almost always lacking in hydrochloric acid. Deficiencies often show up in people age forty and over, but even teenagers show deficiencies as a result of poor diet.

Bulk Up Your Diet . . . .

Fiber is an essential ingredient for a well-functioning liver; it's the garbage truck that carries away cholesterol. White bread, pasta and cereal has had this important fiber removed from the grain. No wonder North Americans

If you're having trouble eliminating, a fiber supplement that includes psyllium husks will add necessary bulk. Be sure to take adequate amounts of water along with it—water is required to make sure that the psyllium husks swell up, and then move out!

worry about high cholesterol! Get back to a daily dietary regimen of whole foods, fruit and vegetables—whole-grain bread, legumes, cooked grains, and raw and steamed vegetables. Emphasize raw foods—up to seventy-five percent. Eating whole and especially raw foods will give you sufficient fiber to facilitate peristaltic movement.

Peristalsis is a series of muscle contractions that moves food and waste along the intestinal tract. Fiber soaks up water ten to thirty times its weight, so you'll need to consume lots of water for proper elimination. Digestion is impeded when too little of either is consumed throughout the day.

The organs work in harmony with every bodily process. Every function is important and affects every other function. When you simply drink water and do not consume fiber-rich food, the water will be expelled through the urinary tract without removing any toxins. Faulty elimination of toxins hampers the bile duct and pancreatic ducts and engorges the liver. The poor pancreas can't supply the digestive juices (enzymes) to the small intestine so that the body can digest food. And when digestion stops so does proper assimilation of food nutrients.

Enzymes

Natural plant enzymes are present in all fruit and vegetables but are destroyed with heat. If you're accustomed to eating mostly cooked food, your pancreas must work harder to supply the enzymes necessary for digestion, which depletes your own store of enzymes. This process accelerates as you get older and your supply of digestive enzymes is reduced year by year. So-o-o, it's vital to take plant enzymes as one of your "supplements" with every cooked meal, as well as tablets of hydrochloric acid with betaine and pepsin.

Yet another problem caused by improper elimination is the probability of parasites. A toxic buildup in the bowel creates an environment conducive for parasites. Parasite incubation time is quick, about thirty-six hours. If you have not eliminated for one, two, three or four days, you may be sure the parasites have moved in—and are cozy and happy!

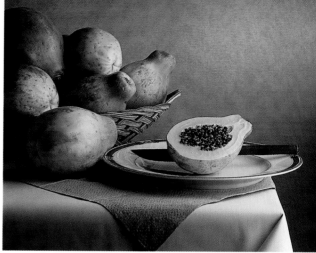

Common wisdom is that bowel elimination should occur after each full meal: three meals daily, three stools; one meal, one stool. If you alter your eating habits to six small meals, eat optimum foods, chew well, and take digestive enzymes with your food, one or two movements a day are enough. The more nutritious the foods, the better the digestive process. Junk food usually doesn't contain the requisite fiber to promote proper peristalsis and as a result, elimination is poor and all the affected organs are stressed.

Weight Loss

The liver is a fat-burning machine and is instrumental in normalizing weight by pumping excess fat out of the body through the bile and into the small intestines. Eating a diet high in fiber reduces the recirculation of fats and other toxins from the gut to the liver. When you eat a low-fiber diet, the bad fats, especially trans-fats and cholesterol, get into the bloodstream; adequate amounts of high-density lipoproteins, or HDL cholesterol (the good kind) are not manufactured; and the bad cholesterol, low-density lipoproteins (LDL) attach to blood vessel walls.

The good fats are natural, freshly pressed oil derived from seeds and nuts such as flax, sunflowers, pumpkin and walnuts, as well as from coconut. These oils provide the essential fatty acids (omega-3 and omega-6) that your body requires and that your liver can easily process in order to maintain a healthy weight. (For more information read *Good Fats and Oils*, *alive* books, 2000)

A roll of fat at the waistline in men or women can be a sign of what is commonly called a "fatty" liver. This is a liver that has stopped processing fat and instead has become a fat-storing organ, engorged and swollen with greasy deposits. No matter how much you exercise, removing this fat "roll" will be impossible until you improve your liver function.

Eliminating this excess fat requires a protocol of detoxification followed by a liver-cleansing regimen. And that takes time and patience. Liver restoration will not happen overnight and may take three to five months or longer. Once the accumulated fat is removed, however, weight loss occurs. You'll feel more alive and "liverish" symptoms will disappear.

Kitchen Wisdom: Foods to Choose . . . .

The liver is very forgiving. The good news is that you don't have to go any farther than your own kitchen to begin detoxifying and improving liver function. It starts with what you choose to eat. Adopting a liver-cleansing diet is relatively easy and painless. It just takes awareness and the will to make a shift in the direction of life and liver enhancement. Food really is your best medicine. Choose the foods your body understands—real food as nature made it—and your digestive and cleansing organs will metabolize efficiently. And efficient metabolism equates to good health.

In order to fulfill the correct process of liver detoxification the nutrients required include:

amino acids	(glutamine, glycine, taurine, cysteine B vitamins)
folic acid	
glutathione	
antioxidants	(carotenoids, vitamins E and C, sulfured phytochemicals in foods such as cruciferous vegetables and garlic)

Vegetables and Fruit

Raw vegetables and fruit are rich in both fiber and water content and are the foundation of sound eating habits. Choose especially the brightly colored foods, like dark green leafy vegetables, tomatoes, red and green peppers, orange squash and yams, red cabbage, purple eggplant, beets, carrots, oranges and papayas. Those bright, rich colors are no accident. They were planned by an intelligent Creator to tempt you to try them, much as the bees are lured to a blossom by scent and a hummingbird by color.

Brightly colored foods contain powerful antioxidants and carotenoids, which are essential nutrients for high performance metabolism and optimum liver function. For instance, tomatoes contain lycopene, an antioxidant considered the most powerful of all the dietary carotenoids. Carrots give you beta-carotene; beet root offers the antioxidant anthocyanidin. Those rich colors translate into rich nutrient value.

If you take these vegetables in the form of freshly pressed juice, your body will quickly absorb the nutrients without the need for long digestion time. (Read *Juicing for the Health of It !* *alive* books, 2000, for more imformation.) Freshly pressed vegetable juice is the best liver-cleansing food and should be part of the daily diet.

Eating fruit and vegetables in their natural raw state, either fresh or juiced, provides the body with specific plant enzymes that promote optimum digestion. When food is cooked these enzymes are destroyed, along with some of the vitamin and mineral content. The digestive system then must work harder to complete the digestive process, placing a strain on other organs, such as the pancreas and liver. So when you do cook vegetables, lightly steam them to preserve as many nutrients as possible. Never overcook.

Freshly pressed vegetable juice is the best liver-cleansing food.

Fats and Oils

Freshly pressed oils, such as flax oil, sunflower seed oil, olive oil and sesame oil are easily emulsified and digested and are essential to building healthy membranes around the liver cells. (Read *Good Fats and Oils, alive* books, 2000, for more information.) Fresh seed and nut oils are, however, damaged by light and heat. Only buy them when they are unrefined and stored in dark glass bottles. And remember to read pressing dates on the bottle labels to determine their freshness. Freshly pressed nut and seed oils can go rancid in a few weeks–and rancid oils are carcinogenic. More toxins for the liver to cope with!

Refined oils have a much longer shelf life, which makes them easy to transport over

Use only unrefined, cold-pressed oils in your kitchen.

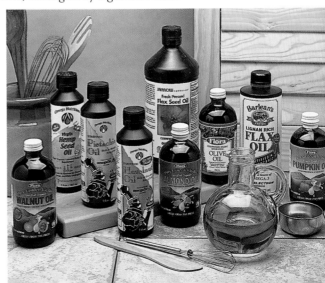

Butter is listed in the good food category. Butter is a natural fat and the liver can handle it in moderation (two to three tablespoons per day).

long distances. However, the high temperatures used in the refining process change the molecular structure of oil and create the very trans-fatty acids that your liver would like you to avoid. If you want to live a long life, eliminate these oils from your diet.

An excellent way to enjoy butter and yet reduce its consumption is to mix soft butter with an equal amount of flax oil, add a sprinkle of finely chopped herbs (basil, parsley or oregano), a little cayenne or garlic and refrigerate. Use this butter-oil mix as a tasty spread for whole-grain bread or crackers, and as a topping for baked potatoes, steamed vegetables and cooked grains.

Fresh, raw nuts and seeds are natural protein foods that the body can assimilate and digest. Remember your body is primitive, not a piece of modern machinery. Nuts and seeds are ancient foods designed for your enjoyment and to nourish and sustain you. However, nature provides them with a protective coating containing enzyme inhibitors to keep them from rotting and the oil from going rancid. (Nuts and seeds will keep for years as long as they're dry.) But the enzyme inhibitors also are hard for human stomachs to digest, so nuts and seeds should be soaked before eating. (Grains and legumes also have enzyme inhibitors. Always soak dried beans, lentils and peas before cooking and discard the soak water).

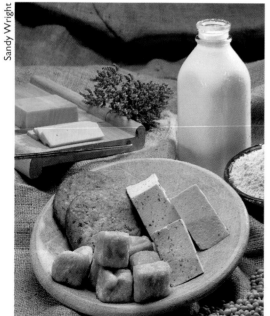

Sandy Wright

Soy—Or No Soy?

Soybeans contain a good source of oil as well as protein. However, all soybean oil has been refined and heat processed. It's not a "natural" choice, no matter what the label says. Soy products have other problems today. Present day soybeans are not the same food that Asians have been eating for generations. Soybean crops are big business and the beans have been hybridized for decades as a normal aspect of plant "science." Add to this the present "science" of altering the bean's intrinsic genes. Now almost all soybeans are genetically engineered and no one knows the long-term effect this will have on human health. Genetically altered food products have not been proven safe and no long-term tests have been done. Your best protection is to look for the certified organic label on all food, including tofu, tempeh and naturally fermented tamari.

Great Grains

Grains, used in various ways, are part of the happy-liver diet. Cooked whole grains, whole-grain bread and crackers are all easy to metabolize for people whose ancestors traditionally made use of these whole foods. People who traditionally did not eat grains as a regular part of their diet can have problems digesting gluten, which is present in most grains, especially wheat. Whole grains, therefore, are recommended for a liver-cleansing diet only for those who have no trouble digesting them. However, when grains are sprouted the gluten is not present; consequently sprouts are usually well tolerated and are good "living" food that promotes healthy liver function.

Eggs—Yes or No?

Eggs are good liver food. A healthy liver can handle up to ten eggs per day, but if you're cleansing, one to three eggs daily is sufficient. Eggs got the bad reputation of being too high in animal fat and therefore high in cholesterol. The public was inundated by an anti-egg message, and before we knew it, everyone accepted as truth that eggs should be avoided. Remember that cholesterol levels in the body are regulated by a healthy liver, not by dietary intake of so-called low-cholesterol or no-cholesterol foods.

Eggs are an excellent source of protein and contain high amounts of lecithin, which has been proven to lower cholesterol. Eggs are also high in the amino acids taurine, cysteine and methionine, all required by the liver to regulate bile production. For optimum metabolism of its nutrients, serve eggs poached or soft-boiled rather than scrambled or in an omelet. Hard-boiled eggs are hard to digest. Avoid cooking eggs until the sulfur in the yolk turns green as they become toxic at this point.

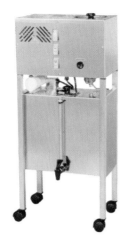

Precision Water Distiller

Good Clean Water

Water helps everything work and is essential for a happy liver. Water as a hydrating, cleansing agent is ideally made up of clean, vibrant, living water molecules that are configured much like snowflakes. Unfortunately, this kind of water is only obtainable in remote, pristine areas of the world, and it definitely does not come out of your city water pipes! Look for steam-distilled water or products from your health food store that will reclaim the life-giving properties of water (see "Sources").

The water from your tap is chlorinated and maybe fluoridated. Both of these substances are toxic gases that the liver must deal with. Don't add them to your liver load!

Foods to Refuse · · · · · · · · · · · · · · · ·

A liver-cleansing diet really involves eating with common sense. Unfortunately, some North Americans have lost that common food sense as a result of modern food processing, marketing methods and advertising.

Non-Food Ingredients

The list of foods to avoid includes all the processed and packaged food products of the giant North American and international food manufacturers. These so-called "foods," so full of non-food ingredients, have become the mainstay of food production at the expense of human health. You need to avoid hydrogenated oils, heat-damaged fats, preservatives, chemical food colors, chemical taste enhancers, pesticides, sugar in all its forms, artificial sweeteners, caffeine and the many non-food additives listed on labels. All of these are liver toxins—yet we still eat them. Your busy liver becomes overworked trying to filter out these poisons so that they do not get into the bloodstream. What a responsibility!

Sweet Treats

Use sweeteners such as honey, maple syrup and sweet, dried fruit only in moderation. Refined sugar is poison. Sweeteners are not part of the regular happy-liver diet no matter how much they tempt your taste buds.

North Americans consume far too much sugar in their diets. Learning to live without sweet foods goes a long way towards keeping your liver happy and healthy. If you make a habit of taking the sugar out when preparing food, even when the recipe calls for it, your taste buds will eventually change for the better.

Dairy Products

Most dairy products—milk, cheese, butter and yogurt—sold in stores today are processed through pasteurization and homogenization and consequently they are no longer whole foods. Choose the European creamery style of butter and some of the famous cheeses from Austria, France, Switzerland and Italy, which are still made from raw, unpasteurized milk. Get in the habit of asking your retailer for unpasteurized products.

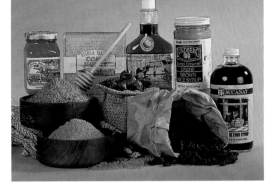

Natural sweeteners include honey, maple syrup, concentrated cane juice (Sucanat® and Rapadura™) and date sugar.

The most ideal sources of milk products are cultured or fermented, in the form of natural buttermilk, yogurt, quark and kefir. These products contain friendly live bacteria and help maintain healthy bacterial flora in the intestines. Look for that live bacteria count on the label of the products you buy, or make your own kefir at home with a handy kefir maker (available at your health food store).

Attitude is Altitude . . . .

Kefir is a popular fermented milk product in many parts of the world, and is now gaining status in the West as a delicious alternative to yogurt. Many of the liver cleansing recipes call for kefir. If you have not yet discovered how easy it is to make kefir, you may substitute with sour cream or crème fraîche.

Consider the liver-cleansing diet an adventure. Embarking on such a diet is like climbing a mountain to see the view from the top—a struggle, but worth the gain in altitude! You'll need careful planning, and most of all, confidence and a positive mind

The wise King Solomon taught that a "merry heart does good like medicine."

set. A positive attitude is very important for a healthy liver, because the liver treats negative emotions such as frustration, anger and hostility as toxins. The liver often cannot deal with these emotional toxins, so they get stored in the muscles and tissues of the body. The result is distress and disease.

Dr E.E. Rogers, a medical maverick who advocated the principles of nutritional healing sixty years ago said, "If you are intelligent enough to eat properly it is better to also like it when you are doing it. The diet will work better if you do the necessary things in the proper spirit!"

Be positive, be grateful for what you have, and enjoy real food. Then your liver will relax and do its job properly.

The Liver Cleanse . . . .

This procedure is sometimes called a liver "flush." It is designed to cleanse the liver of toxins, fat and sludge and to flush out the "stones" of fatty and calcified deposits that we call gall stones. The longer bile remains in the gallbladder the thicker this bitter, greenish liquid becomes and the greater the likelihood of stones forming. These stones also form when too little bile is produced. They in turn decrease the ability of the liver to make bile and as a result, less cholesterol and toxins are removed from the body.

Essential fatty acids (from sources such as flax seed oil and evening primrose oil) stimulate bile production and help transport cholesterol and fatty sludge out of the liver. When you get rid of gallstones, digestion improves dramatically, allergies go away and back pain disappears! It seems

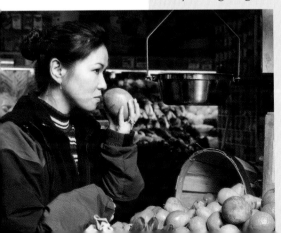

like a miracle. It's not. It's just a greatly relieved liver that is now able to move toxins out.

I don't recommend jumping into a liver flush unless you have been on the liver-cleansing diet for at least a few weeks. And ideally the liver flush itself requires dietary preparation for one or two days in advance: eat only raw foods and drink eight to ten glasses of freshly pressed vegetable juice and at least eight glasses of water daily. This cleansing regimen facilitates the procedure and lessens the chance of a bad reaction, such as nausea or vomiting. If you are nervous about doing it, you probably shouldn't. Again, attitude and confidence are important.

Perform the liver flush on a weekend when you have time to keep to the protocol, to rest and to get to the bathroom quickly when necessary. Get up bright and early, go for a long walk and do deep breathing exercises to oxygenate the tissues and relax any tension. Continue to drink water throughout the day.

There are many recipes for flushing the liver and gallbladder. Any regimen that makes use of the cleansing properties of lemon, garlic, cayenne and olive oil will work more or less. The following is one method I've found successful when I faithfully adhere to the protocol.

Squeeze enough grapefruit, lemons or limes to make eleven ounces (300 ml) of juice. Dilute with seven ounces (200 ml) steam-distilled water (filtered water will also do).

Chop one or two cloves of fresh garlic and half a teaspoon of fresh ginger root then press both together in a garlic press to release the juices. You can also use half a teaspoon of cayenne in place of the ginger. Add the pressed garlic and ginger to the water and juice mixture.

Pour eleven ounces (300 ml) of extra-virgin olive oil into a warm glass.

The procedure is to swallow three tablespoons of the juice mixture and three tablespoons of the olive oil every fifteen minutes, relaxing between doses by lying down with a hot-water bottle over the liver area. This moist heat dilates the bile ducts and helps to release small stones and sludge from the gallbladder. You could also sit in a warm bath, but I find the hot-water bottle method easier to do.

The whole process can take some hours, so turn off the telephone and be patient. Enjoy the fact that you're doing something wonderful for your liver and thus your whole body. Bowel elimination will start to happen along with some possible discomfort and cramping. Don't worry. Sing a song. Massage your abdomen, following the line of the ascending, transverse and descending colon. Sip fresh water, breathe deeply and relax if you feel nauseous.

If you're stout-hearted and curious you can empty your bowels in a bucket in order to count the small, greenish stones or grit that you pass with every movement. Some of them may be no bigger than a small pea, some may be large and soft, full of fatty sludge (cholesterol). Be happy that you're getting rid of them. And if you stay on a liver-cleansing diet, you may not make any more. A healthy liver manufactures and secretes healthy bile, which prevents gallbladder inflammation and the formation of stones.

The day after the flush, stay on your liver-cleansing diet of freshly pressed vegetable juice, raw fruit and vegetables, and steamed and baked vegetables. Eat moderately and exercise.

Liver-Loving Herbs . . . .

The liver loves bitters. People have long used bitter herbs for liver cleansing, especially after a long winter. Wild herbs such as dandelion greens, endive, artichoke, onion, garlic, radicchio and lettuce, were harvested and dried for later use.

All bitter herbs aid liver function and encourage the secretion of bile. Unfortunately, our cultivated herbs have had the "bitters" bred out of most varieties through hybridizing: the popular iceberg lettuce, for instance, is devoid of any nutrients, but it has a long shelf life! Because of modern marketing and availability, you've learned to like iceberg lettuce and hate bitters. But your body needs bitters, and herbs are now the best source of them.

Medicinal Herbs

Herbs that are specific for cleansing the liver include golden seal, wormwood, rue, celandine and milk thistle. Herbs are synergistic, that is, they help one another in function. Medicinal herbs are best taken in compatible combination and for periods of time only. Thus you should adhere to a protocol for three to six weeks or vary some combinations daily, according to need.

Herbs come in capsule form or can be taken as a tea infusion that you sip throughout the day. The age-old recipe for Swedish bitters, for instance, is a combination of eleven herbs that has been used effectively for hundreds of years. You can buy Swedish bitters at your health food store or get the dried herbs and brew your own.

Make an infusion by pouring boiling water over the leaves and blossoms and steeping for five minutes or more before drinking. Berries can be steeped the same way, but roots and bark should be simmered from five to fifteen minutes to release their active ingredients. In the case of a herbal combination of roots, bark, berries and leaves you can powder them in a spice mill or coffee grinder and take the powdered mixture in a capsule or teaspoon, or pour boiling water over the mixture.

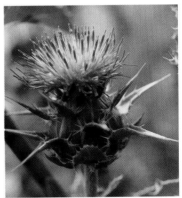

Milk thistle

Natural medicinal plant juices are also available in health food stores. Those specific for the liver are dandelion juice, nettle juice and black radish juice. Artichoke is a member of the thistle family and a natural liver tonic: it stimulates the production and the flow of bile and aids in the process of detoxification.

Make liver herbs a regular part of your liver-friendly regimen, and especially take a combination of liver herbs whenever you feel sluggish, the morning after overeating, over-drinking or when you feel depressed, fatigued or aching.

For instance, fennel seed, anise, ginger, peppermint and licorice root make infusions (tea) that are pleasant to taste and soothing to

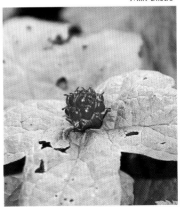

Logan berry

digest. Use one of them as your "taste enhancer" along with three or four bitter herbs. These herbs are available in most health food stores and can be made into a tea. Don't add sweetener. Just take the tea like the medicine it is! Herbs that help the liver are almost all bitter, that's why they're effective in detoxification. Taking them with an aromatic herb will help the medicine go down.

Bitter Herbs and Their Friends	
• barberry (Barberis vulgaris)*	• anise (Pimpinella anisum)
• fennel seed (Foeniculum vulgare)	• lobelia (Lobelia inflata)
• wild yam (Dioscorea villosa)	• marshmallow root (Althea officinalis)
• ginger (Zingiber officinalis)	• skullcap (Scutellaria lateriflora)*
• catnip (Nepeta cataria)	• walnut bark (Juglans nigra)*
• peppermint (Mentha piperita)	• cayenne (Capsicum frutescens)
• gravel root (Eupatorium purpureum)	• golden seal (Hydrastis Canadensis)*
• licorice root (Glycyrrhiza glabra)	• wormwood (Artemisia absintheum)*
• milk thistle (Silybum marianum)*	• rue (Ruta graveolens)

bitter herbs

Culinary Herbs

Fresh herbs will keep for a few weeks in the refrigerator when wrapped in a damp paper towel and then placed in plastic wrap or a container.

The use of herbs in cooking is gaining popularity as cooks discover the wonderful qualities of these common plants. Culinary herbs are the most ancient and increasingly the most popular taste enhancers, since they come from nature's bounty and not from the chemist's laboratory. Using fresh herbs are always best and they are now readily available, even in winter. There's a nutritional as well as a flavor benefit from the "vital" or life force of the fresh plant compared to the dried herbs that have sat on your spice rack for years!

The custom in East Indian households is to put herb seeds such as dill, caraway and anise on the dining table to chew along with meals as digestive aids. Peppermint is also soothing to both the stomach and digestive tract.

To help you season your dishes for optimum taste enhancement, here are a few harmonious vegetable and herb combinations.

Seasoning Suggestions
- beets: basil, bay leaf, cardamom, dill, tarragon broccoli marjoram, oregano, tarragon
- Brussels sprouts: basil, dill, caraway, savory, thyme
- carrots: basil, dill, marjoram, parsley, thyme
- cauliflower: dill, rosemary, summer savory, tarragon

- cabbage: caraway, celery seed, dill, summer savory, tarragon
- cucumber: basil, savory tarragon
- green beans: basil, dill, rosemary, thyme, oregano
- onions: basil, oregano, thyme
- peas: basil, dill, mint, oregano
- potatoes: basil, chives, dill, marjoram, mint, parsley
- squash: basil, dill, oregano, savory
- spinach: rosemary, oregano, tarragon
- tomatoes: basil, bay leaf, parsley, oregano

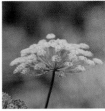

Dill

Use herbs generously and creatively when preparing your meals. In addition to tasting great, herbs contribute to your overall well-being. The liver-cleansing lifestyle is a commitment to health and longevity and herbs help you build a healthy liver for optimum living.

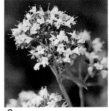

Celandine

Planning the Liver-Cleansing Menu . . . .

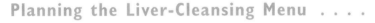

For most people, planning daily meals requires a firm reign on normal habits. Write down your particular dietary goals. It will be easier to stick with them when you read them over every day.

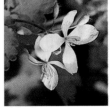

Oregano

Fresh Vegetable Juice

A healthy liver is the result of a regular diet of nutrient-dense foods. Vegetables are both cleansing and building to the liver, and in the form of freshly pressed vegetable juice are easy to digest and quickly deliver a whole lot of vitamins and minerals to your body.

Make sure you drink at least eight ounces (240 ml) of freshly pressed juice daily. You should actually "chew" your vegetable juice in order to stimulate salivary glands and start the digestive process. The more you include vegetable juice in your diet the easier it is on your liver.

Carrot, beet, spinach, celery, cabbage, cucumber–they all juice well and can be used in various combinations. My favorite mix is carrot, celery and apple with a little ginger for extra flavor and for its liver-loving properties. But since I regard freshly pressed juice as medicine as well as food I include some bitter greens: dandelion leaves, endive, radicchio. Radish is also an excellent liver stimulant for its sharp, biting flavor, especially

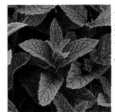

Mint

Sandy Wright

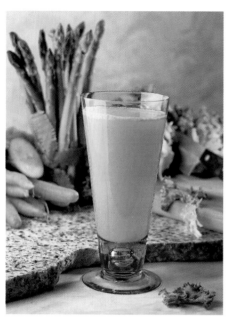

black radish. And I make a point of adding beet root to my juice regularly. It's an ideal blood cleanser.

I mention a compatible combination in the recipe section to get you started if juicing is new to you, but you can create your own combinations according to what you like, what's available and what you are aware will facilitate the cleansing process. Spinach, lettuce, radish and cabbage are all juiceable. Wild greens are available to many people and include dandelion, pigweed and lamb's quarters, as long as you're sure they have not been sprayed with pesticides.

Juicing three times a day is suggested if you have the time. (If you have a Green Power juicer you can juice once to provide enough juice for the whole day. The magnets in the juice-extracting system prevent oxidization of fruit and vegetables.) Make the regimen fit your lifestyle, but adjust your lifestyle to what is best for your liver.

Breakfast

Your body has properly fasted since the last meal at six the night before. Your liver has been able to complete its task of detoxification during the night and you wake refreshed. You bounce out of bed! The nourishment the liver likes at this point is the juice of half a lemon in a glass of distilled water followed by two or three more glasses of water and maybe a cup of liver-cleansing tea–without sweetener. Then take a brisk walk for an hour. Or perhaps spend half an hour on the exercise machine and a half-hour jogging. In the summer, weed the garden; in the winter spend an hour in the local pool or gym. I prefer walking in the fresh air all year long no matter the weather.

By this time you've earned your first meal. Make it light. Have your fresh vegetable juice now. Or a fresh grapefruit or other fruit, with more fruit mid-morning. But if you need something more substantial this is a good time to enjoy a dish of muesli or cooked cereal of oatmeal, millet, buckwheat or brown rice. This is also when some like to have a soft-boiled egg or two. Take a digestive enzyme with cooked food.

Mid-Day Meal

If you're at home you have opportunity to prepare this most important meal. If at work you will probably have to prepare in advance and carry food with you. Bring fresh ingredients for a salad, along with some pre-cooked grain and a little last minute fixings in the staff lunchroom.

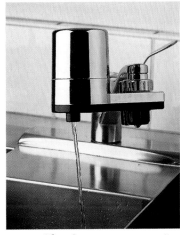

water filter

The noon meal should be unhurried and relaxed. Avoid eating a quick, light lunch, stuffing yourself at the dinner table, and then going to bed full.

Main Dishes

For most people the evening is set aside for the main meal, a time when all the family is home and can cook and share food together. You need to accompany your main dish with a raw salad of greens or grated root vegetables. Remember, at least seventy-five percent of your diet should be raw.

Adhere to the liver-cleansing diet for a minimum of twenty-one days and more preferably for a full three months to you really experience the benefits. After that you may feel so fit you'll want to stay with it!

Once your liver is grooving along, it will let you know and you won't want to go back to feeling sluggish. With a few pardonable indulgences along the way, liver cleansing will be a way of life!

Muesli is an uncooked grain-and-fruit breakfast (traditionally made with soaked oat flakes and grated apple) that is popular with many Europeans. North Americans are learning to love it. Make your own muesli rather than buying the pre-packaged variety from the supermarket. Muesli is not restricted to breakfast, however. It's a wholesome snack any time of day and it could even be a lunch-box meal. Follow my suggestions for making homemade muesli in the recipe section (page 32), or you can create your own with oats, chopped nuts, berries, peaches and grated apple, and add lemon juice and kefir, yogurt or nut milk to moisten.

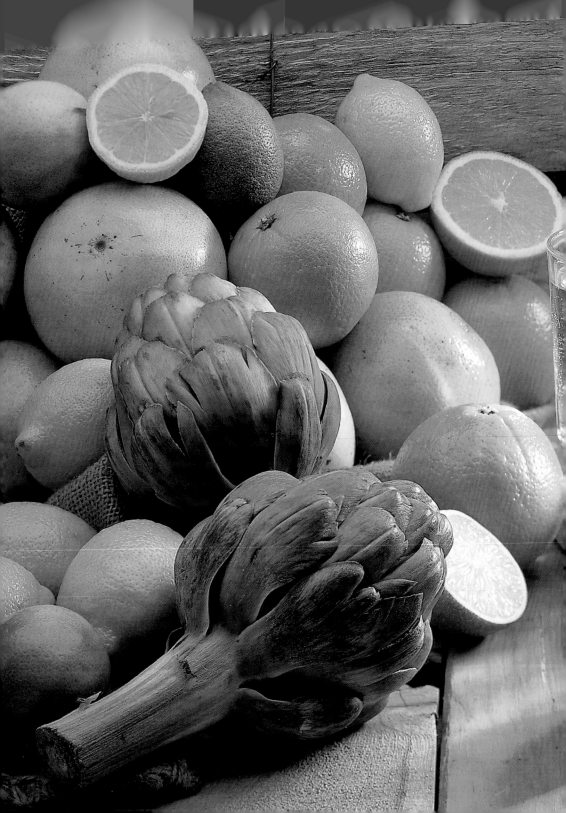

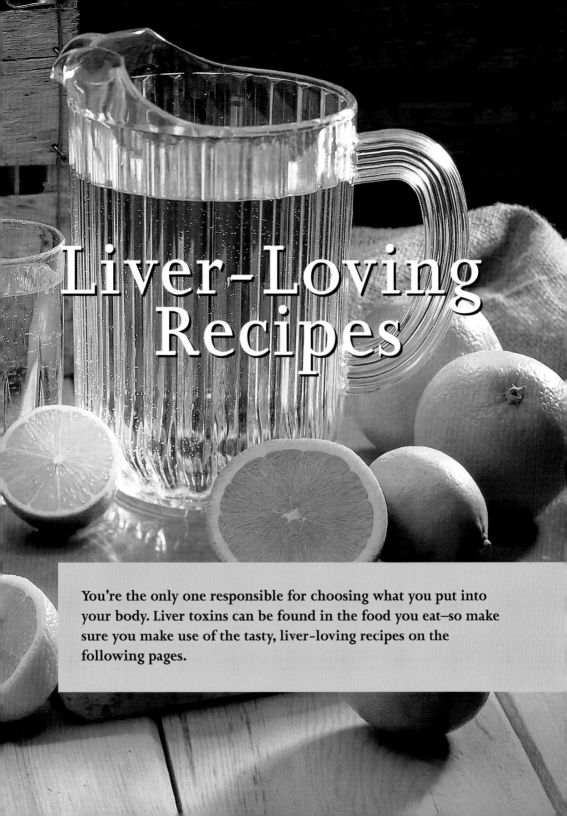

Liver-Loving Recipes

You're the only one responsible for choosing what you put into your body. Liver toxins can be found in the food you eat–so make sure you make use of the tasty, liver-loving recipes on the following pages.

Banana-Apple Muesli

This combination of fruit, nuts and wheat germ supplies an abundance of vitamin B, calcium, phosphorus, iron and potassium.

½ **cup (125 ml) kefir**

1 tbsp honey

1 medium-size apple

Juice of 1 lemon

1 medium-size banana

3 tbsp wheat germ

2 or more freshly shelled walnuts

Mix the kefir with the honey until smooth. Peel and core the apple and grate it into the kefir. Immediately add lemon juice so the apple does not oxidize. Peel and slice the bananas into small pieces and mix it with the wheat germ. Fold the bananas and wheat germ into the kefir then serve, garnished with walnuts, in two small bowls.

Serves 2

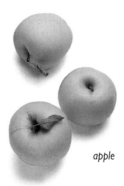

apple

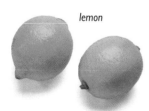

lemon

Eating kefir or yogurt regularly provides the friendly bacteria that will help digestion.

Be sure to purchase wheat germ from the frozen food section of the health food store and remember, the oil in wheat germ goes rancid quickly, so use it up.

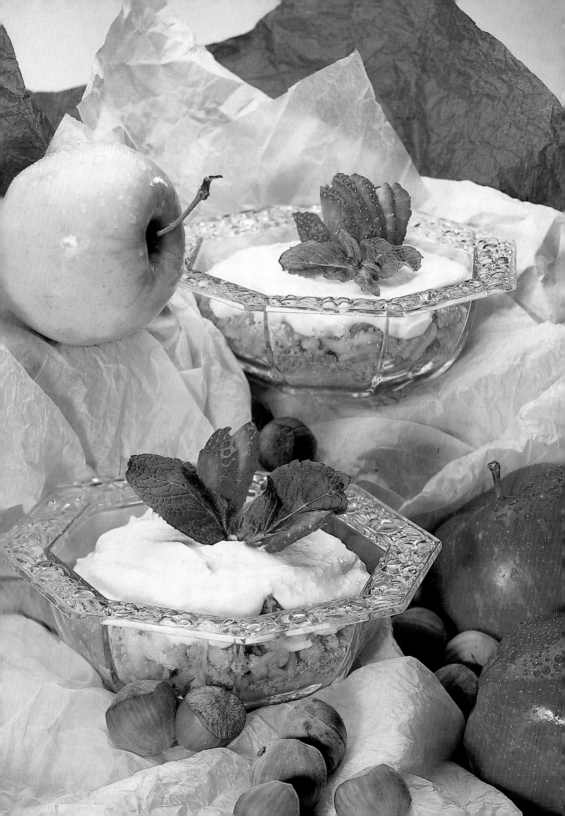

Bircher–Muesli with Sesame Seeds

Treat yourself with this gourmet muesli and remember to eat slowly, savor the flavor and chew well. Sesame seeds are rich in calcium, unsaturated fatty acids, vitamins and minerals, and have been used extensively for thousands of years in India, China, Mexico and Ethiopia. Seeds are preferably not heated, since heat damages the oil in the seed, but roasted sesame does have a wonderful flavor! So take your choice.

4 tsp sesame seeds

1 tsp raisins

⅓ cup (80 g) rolled oats, soaked overnight or at least 1 hour

2 tbsp maple syrup

2 medium-size bananas

½ cup (125 ml) kefir

3 tbsp wheat germ

Soak the raisins and rolled oats in lukewarm water, preferably overnight, or for at least 10 minutes.

In a saucepan, gently brown the sesame seeds. Add the rolled oats, maple syrup and finely sliced bananas to the kefir. Drain raisins. Add wheat germ and raisins to the kefir and mix thoroughly. Sprinkle roasted sesame seeds over top of the muesli just before serving.

Serves 2

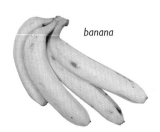

banana

Flax seeds–ground but not heated–may be used in place of sesame seeds, if you wish.

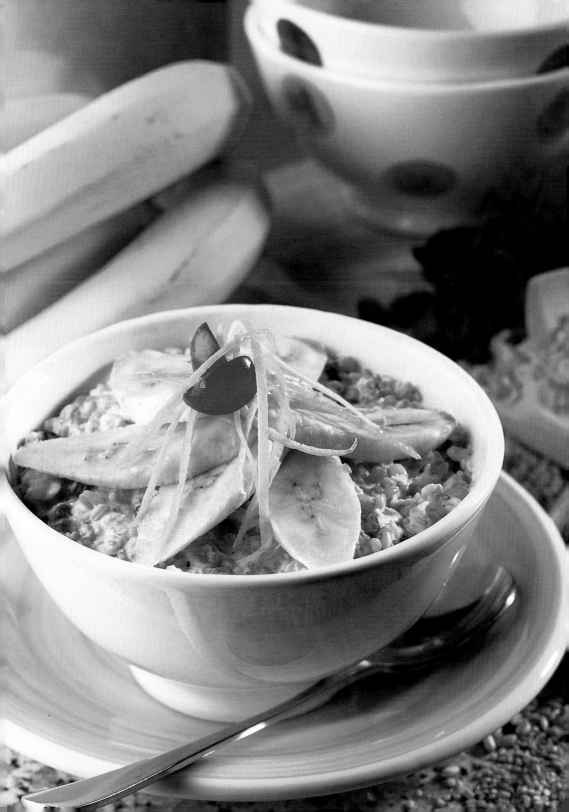

Avocado Duo with Carrots and Beets

This "living" lunch looks and tastes delicious and is quick to make.

2 carrots, freshly grated

2 medium-size beets, freshly grated

I stalk celery, chopped

5-6 red onion rings

I avocado, halved

Grapefruit segments for garnish

2 slices lemon for garnish

Dressing:

I tbsp fresh parsley and mint, finely chopped

3 tbsp flax seed oil

Juice of half a lemon

Tamari soy sauce

Dressing Variation:

I½ cups (375 ml) **kefir**

2 tbsp flax seed oil

Juice of half a lemon

I tsp cumin, freshly ground

Fresh cilantro, finely chopped

Mix together all the dressing ingredients. Toss carrots, beets, celery and onion in the dressing (don't allow the carrots to oxidize). Serve on avocado halves garnished with grapefruit sections and a slice of lemon.

Serves 2

red onion

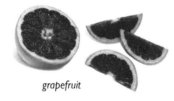

grapefruit

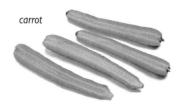

carrot

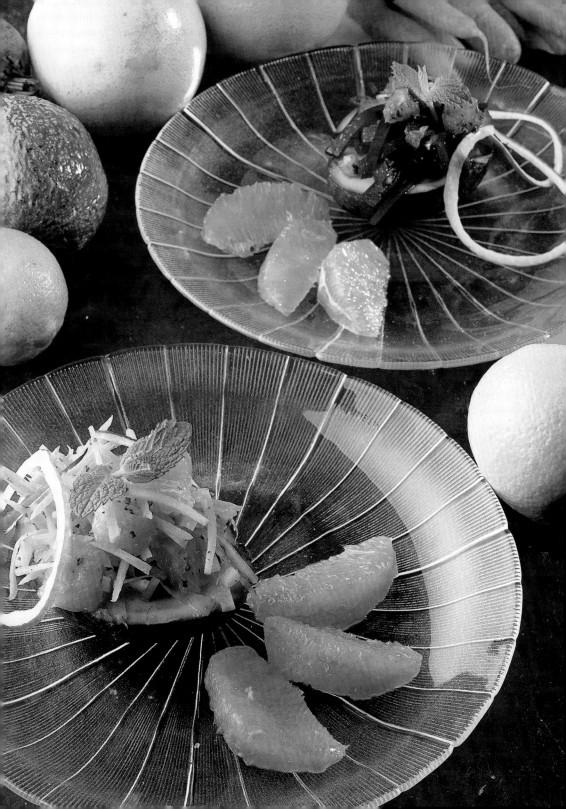

Mediterranean Bread Salad

This is a tasty sandwich substitute. The herb-kefir dressing helps blend the flavors of the rye bread and vegetables.

¼ **cup (100 g) raisins, soaked**

1 long English cucumber, sliced diagonally

4 thick slices heavy rye bread, cut in chunks

½ **cup (125 ml) kefir or yogurt to taste**

1½ **tsp chopped fresh dill, or to taste**

Juice of half a lemon, or to taste

Freshly shelled walnuts, halved

Lime slices for garnish

Soak the raisins in lukewarm water for at least 10 minutes.

Drain the raisins and place them in a large bowl with the cucumber and rye bread. Mix together the kefir, dill and lemon juice and then pour over the cucumber and bread. Serve with walnut halves and a garnish of lime.

Serves 2

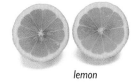

lemon

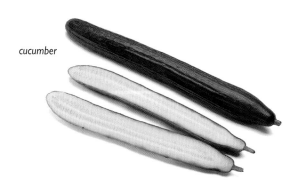

cucumber

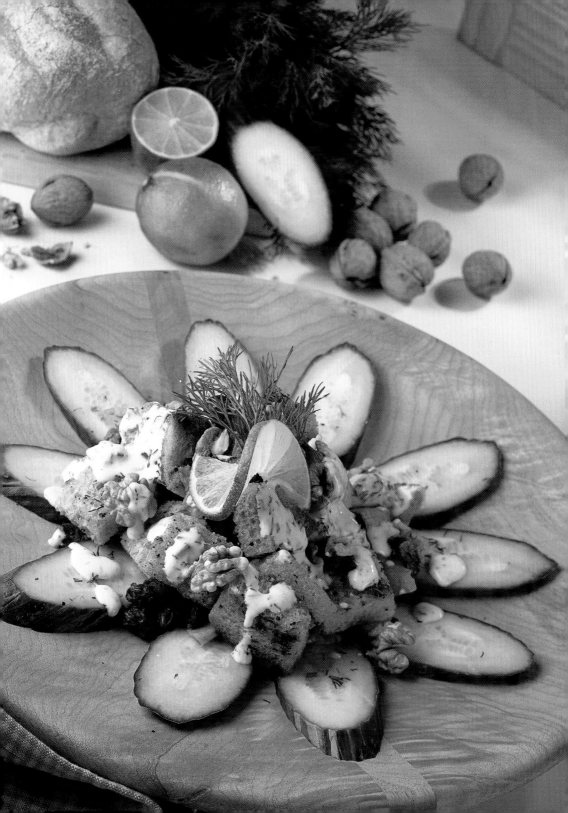

Tofu and Salad Greens

I love eating firm tofu, cubed and marinated in tamari. This recipe makes a substantial meal, especially if you treat yourself to a second helping.

1 block firm tofu (certified organic)**, cut in cubes**

2 medium-size tomatoes, chopped

2 green onions, chopped

½-1 cup (100-200 g) **alfalfa sprouts**

6 mushrooms, sliced

10 edible pea pods, sliced

2 stalks celery, chopped

6 cauliflower florets, blanched in hot water for 2 minutes

Mixed organic salad greens

Ruby red grapefruit segments

Marinate the tofu overnight for at least 2 hours.

Place the dressing ingredients in a jar and shake well. In a large bowl, toss the salad ingredients, except greens, with the dressing so that the pieces are well coated. Add the marinated tofu. Serve on mixed greens with sections of ruby red grapefruit on the side.

Serves 2

Marinade for tofu:

¼ cup (60 ml) **tamari soy sauce**

2 tsp toasted sesame oil

1 tsp lemon juice

Pinch of cayenne pepper

Dressing:

¼ cup (60 ml) **blended cold-pressed oil** (flax, sunflower, olive, safflower and/or sesame)

Juice of half a lemon

Dash of tamari soy sauce

Pinch of cayenne pepper

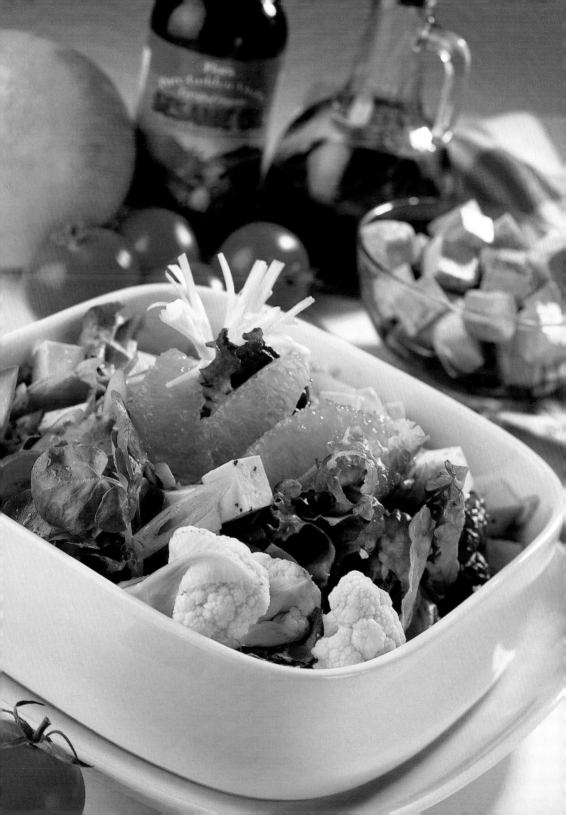

Colorful Cabbage Salad

Cabbage is one of the most versatile vegetables. It tastes great cooked or raw, and is rich in vitamins and minerals. Enjoy this grated salad in summer or winter.

½ **small green cabbage, julienned**

½ **small red cabbage, julienned**

½ **yellow pepper, julienned**

½ **red pepper, julienned**

½ **medium-size red onion, julienned**

½ **cup** (125 g) **fresh pineapple, chopped**

½ **cup** (125 g) **fresh raw corn kernels**

Finely chopped fresh parsley, to taste

Finely chopped fresh mint, to taste

2 large cabbage leaves

Strips of red and yellow pepper for garnish

Place the dressing ingredients in a jar and shake well. Blanche the cabbage in boiling water for 30 seconds. Toss the cabbage and the remaining salad ingredients with the dressing. Serve in a fresh cabbage leaf cup garnished with strips of red and yellow pepper.

Serves 2

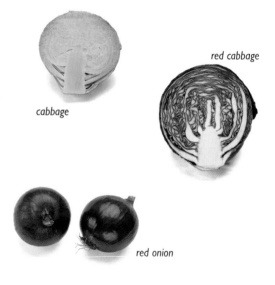

red cabbage

cabbage

red onion

Dressing:

½ **cup** (125 ml) **cold-pressed walnut, hazelnut or flax oil**

1 tbsp apple cider vinegar

Juice of one lemon

Freshly ground anise, to taste

Dill seed, to taste

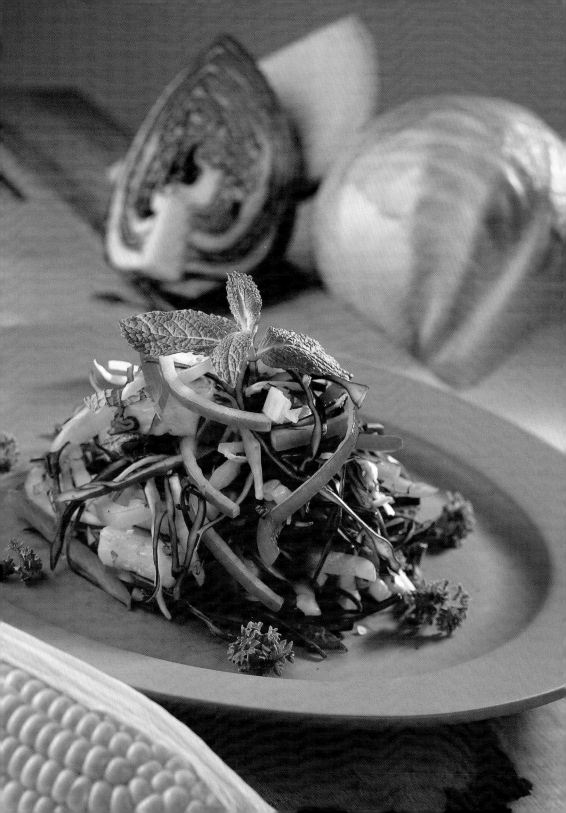

Endive Salad with Potato

A tangy potato dressing accompanies the liver-loving endive in an unusual and hearty combination. Your guests will love it. The original recipe calls for sour cream or cream, but I've substituted kefir, which is less rich and easier to digest. If you are not lactose intolerant, however, try using the cream. I like this dressing both ways.

2 large Yukon Gold potatoes

½ bunch parsley, finely chopped

1 large tomato, cut in sections

1 small head endive, divided into leaves

8 cherry tomatoes

Dressing:

2 tbsp freshly pressed flax seed oil

½ tsp Dijon mustard

6-8 tbsp kefir

Juice of half a lemon

Dash of sea salt

Steam the potatoes in the skin until tender and then peel (if you wish) and slice. Set some parsley aside for garnish. Combine potatoes, tomato sections and the rest of the parsley.

Mix together the dressing ingredients and toss with the potatoes and tomatoes. Divide the endive leaves onto two plates, place the potato mixture over top, then serve garnished with cherry tomatoes and parsley.

Serves 2

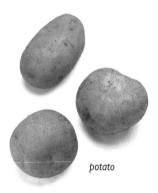

potato

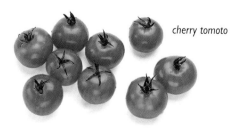

cherry tomoto

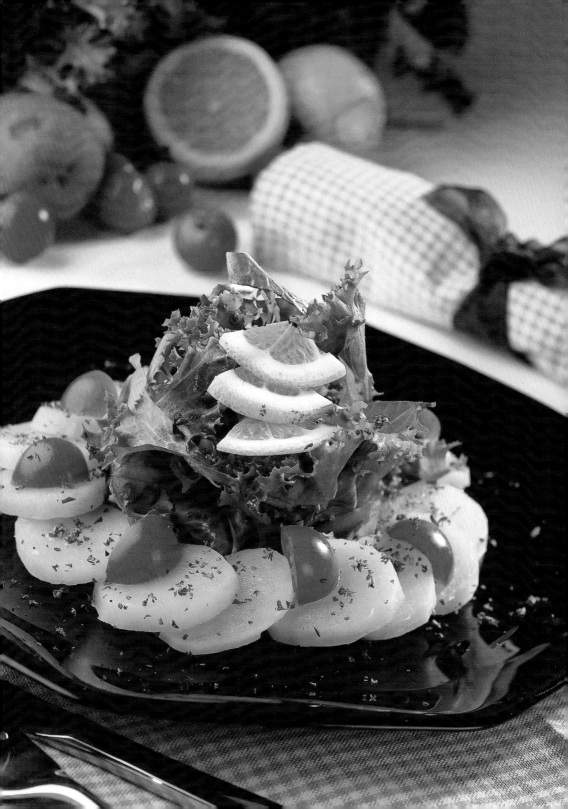

Waldorf Salad

This traditional Waldorf salad is full of minerals and vitamins: calcium, potassium, magnesium, iron, and vitamins B, C and E. The celery root (celeriac) is especially good for the liver.

1 tbsp lemon juice

¼ cup (100 g) chopped walnuts or cashews

½ cup (150 ml) kefir or yogurt

2 tbsp Sultana raisins, soaked

1 cup (220 g) celeriac, peeled and julienned

2 medium-size apples, cubed

2 large leaves butter lettuce

Watercress for garnish

Soak the raisins in lukewarm water for at least 10 minutes.

Mix together the nut cream, lemon juice and chopped nuts. Drain the raisins and add them, along with the kefir, celeriac and apples, to the nut cream. Place a crisp lettuce leaf on each of the two plates, fill with the salad and serve garnished with watercress.

Serves 2

Nut cream:

Put nuts in the blender along with sufficient water to cover. Blend until the mixture is thick with a smooth and creamy consistency.

This recipe originally called for cream or crème fraîche. Suit yourself. It's great with Kefir or cream.

Assorted Vegetable with Frisée

¼ cup grapes

1 cup frisée salad

4-5 cherry tomatoes

2-3 baby carrots, peeled

½ cup baby spinach leafs

½ cup romaine lettuce

½ cup sliced apples

This delicious recipe is featured on the cover of this book.

Dressing:

2 tbsp lemon juice

2 tbsp walnut or flax oil

1 tsp maple syrup

salt & pepper, to taste

Wash all vegetables and lettuce. Toss all ingredients with your dressing, place on a plate and garnish with cherry tomatoes. You can serve this with a freshly baked whole wheat baguette.

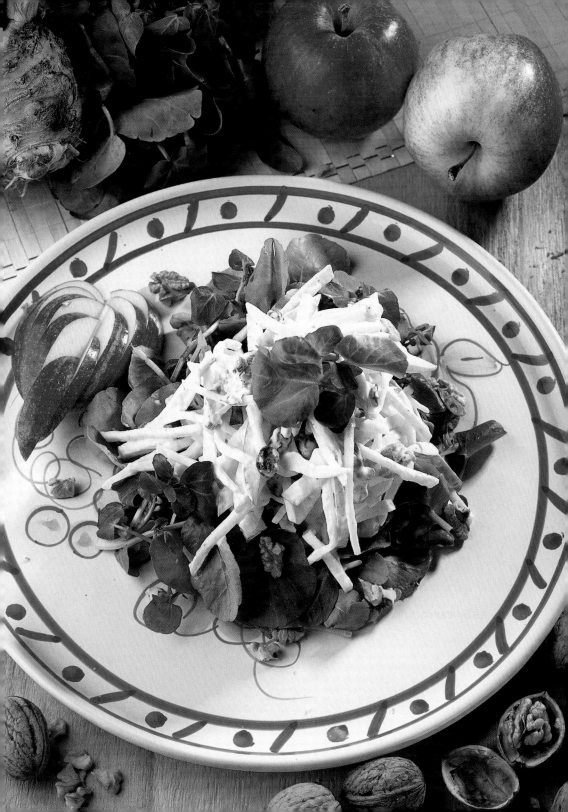

Ratatouille

Serve this cooked dish with steamed brown rice, millet or steamed potatoes and grated Parmesan cheese, accompanied by a raw salad of greens or grated root vegetables. That's a complete meal!

2 tbsp extra-virgin olive oil

1 medium-size red onion, finely chopped

4 cloves garlic, minced

2 medium-size carrots

3 stalks celery

1 yellow pepper

1 red pepper

4 medium-size beefsteak tomatoes

2 small zucchinis

1 medium-size eggplant

1 tsp tomato paste

Fresh parsley, chopped

1 sprig each of fresh thyme, marjoram, tarragon and sage

1 bay leaf

Pinch of sea salt

½ tsp turmeric powder

Cut the vegetables into chunks. In a stainless steel frying pan or wok, heat the olive oil over low heat (never let oil smoke) then sauté the onions and garlic for 2 or 3 minutes. Add the vegetables separately: carrots, then celery, peppers, tomatoes, zucchinis and eggplant last. Vegetables should be crisp. Add tomato paste, herbs and salt. Sprinkle with parsley just before serving.

Serves 2

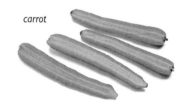

carrot

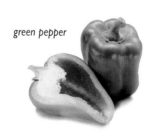

green pepper

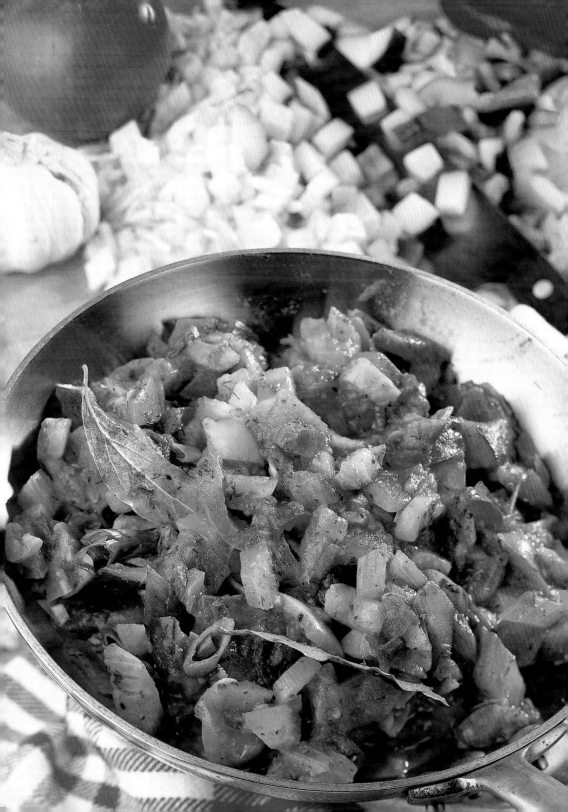

Irish Colcannon

The name for this traditional Irish dish comes from the Gaelic word meaning "white-headed cabbage." If you don't eat eggs or cheese you can leave them out–that's how the Irish served this dish.

6 medium-size potatoes

¼ cup (60 g) butter

I tsp sea salt

⅛ tsp cayenne pepper, or to taste

½ cup (60 ml) nut milk or unhomogenized cow's milk

I ½ cups (300 g) shredded green cabbage

I cup (250 g) finely chopped leeks

¼ cup (60 ml) fine dry whole-grain bread crumbs

¼ cup (60 g) freshly grated Gouda cheese

2 eggs

Preheat the oven to 350°F (190°C).

Scrub and then cook the potatoes in a small amount of water (reserve the liquid) then mash them by hand, leaving the skin on (don't use the food processor). Add 1 tablespoon of butter and the salt, cayenne and milk, then mix thoroughly. Cook the cabbage in the potato water for about 5 minutes.

In the meantime, gently sauté the leeks in a tablespoon of the butter until soft. Strain the cabbage. In a large bowl mix together the potatoes, cabbage and leeks. Butter a 1½ quart (1½ liter) baking dish, sprinkle with bread crumbs and spoon the mixture into the dish. Sprinkle the remaining bread crumbs over top, then dot with the last 2 tablespoons of butter and sprinkle with the grated cheese. Bake in the oven for about 20 minutes and serve immediately.

Serves 2

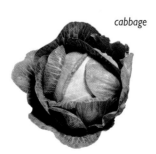

cabbage

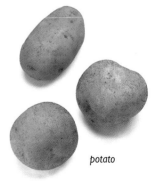

potato

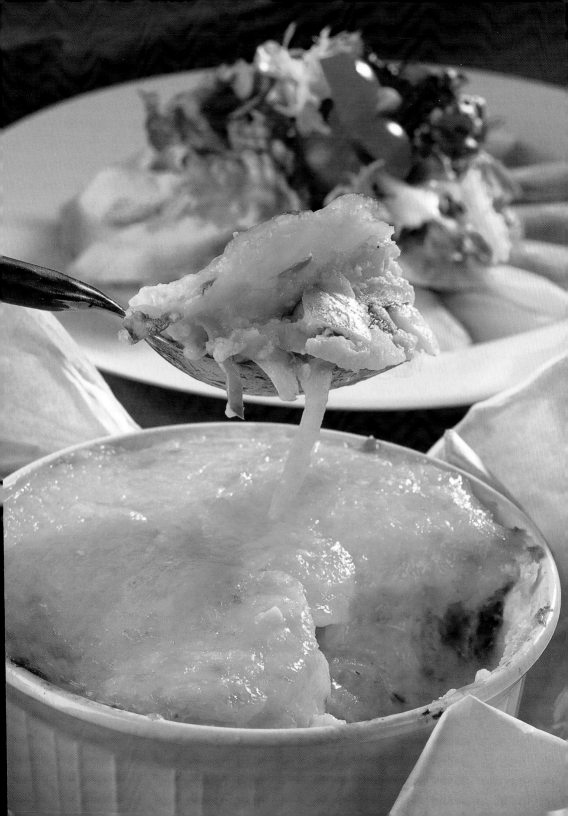

Yam and Parsnip Curry

The orange yams and white parsnips make a colorful and wonderfully tasty dish that is good enough to serve at a party. You can also experiment with squash, pumpkin or zucchini. Serve this curry dish by itself, with a small green salad, a serving of basmati or jasmine rice or a side dish of papaya adds just the right tropical taste.

⅔ cup (150 g) butter

1 tbsp turmeric powder

2 tbsp freshly ground coriander

2 tbsp freshly ground cumin

½ tsp cayenne pepper, or to taste

1 tsp sea salt

3 cups (450 g) chopped leeks

⅓ cup (100 g) grated fresh ginger

8 cups (1.5 kg) parsnips, cut in chunks

10 cups (2 kg) yam, cut in chunks

3 cups (750 ml) water

In a large pot, gently sauté the spices and salt in butter for 1 minute. Add leeks and ginger and sauté for a few more minutes, then add the parsnips and 1 cup of water. Simmer for 6 minutes then add the yams and remaining water. Simmer 6 minutes more, or until yams are tender, stirring occasionally to prevent sticking.

Serves 12

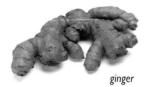

ginger

If you don't have the individual curry spices on hand, substitute them with Bengal or Madras curry powder.

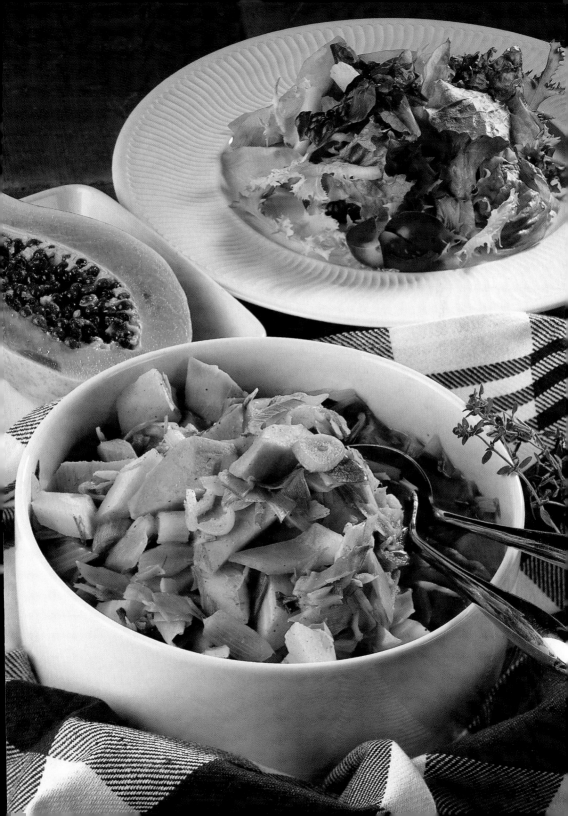

Pumpkin-Broccoli Pot

This wonderfully warming dish will satisfy two hungry people when served with cooked millet or buckwheat.

½ **tbsp extra-virgin olive oil**

I cup (300 g) **pumpkin, cut in chunks**

2 cups (400 g) **broccoli, chopped**

½ **tsp dill weed**

I tbsp lemon juice

I cup water

Sea salt and freshly ground pepper to taste

¼ **cup** (60 ml) **kefir**

In a large saucepan, heat the olive oil over low heat and gently sauté the pumpkin for 3 to 4 minutes. Add broccoli, dill weed, lemon juice, seasoning and just enough water to steam the broccoli until tender but still bright green. Don't overcook. Stir in the kefir and serve.

Serves 2

broccoli

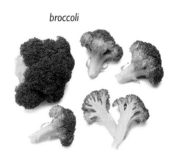

pumpkin

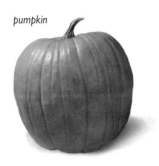

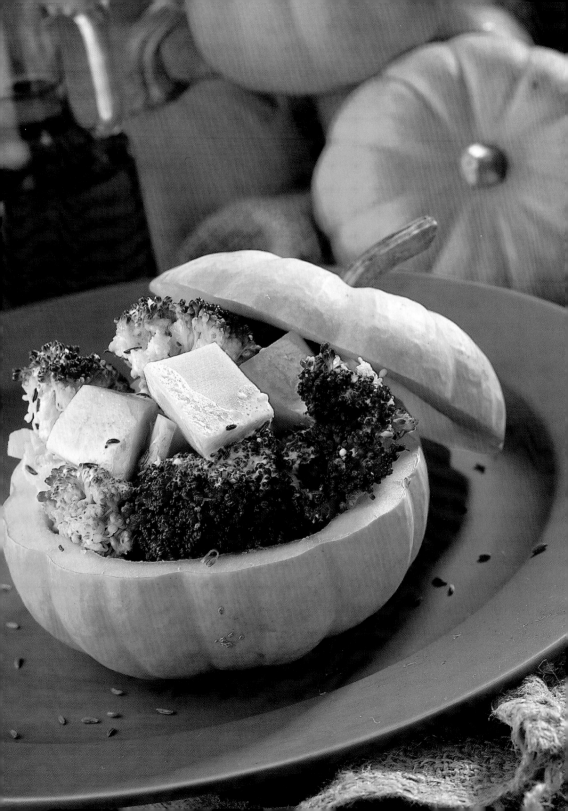

Tomato/Broccoli Simmer

This dish is hearty enough to eat on its own, but I like it best served over rice or quinoa.

1 tbsp extra-virgin olive oil

1 small shallot, minced

2 cloves garlic, minced

2 cups (600 g) broccoli tops and stems

fresh basil, chopped

fresh oregano, chopped

Pinch of cayenne pepper

1 tsp lemon juice

1 cup (250 g) tomatoes, chopped

10 black olives, sliced

In a large pot, heat the olive oil over low heat and gently sauté the shallots and garlic. Add the broccoli, herbs and lemon juice and simmer, covered, for 5 minutes, then add the tomatoes. Stir in the black olives when the vegetables are just tender and serve.

Serves 2

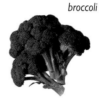

broccoli

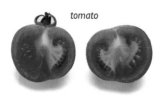

tomato

Putting a little water in the pan before you heat up olive oil prevents the oil from getting too hot. I sometimes like to eliminate the oil and sauté in water only.

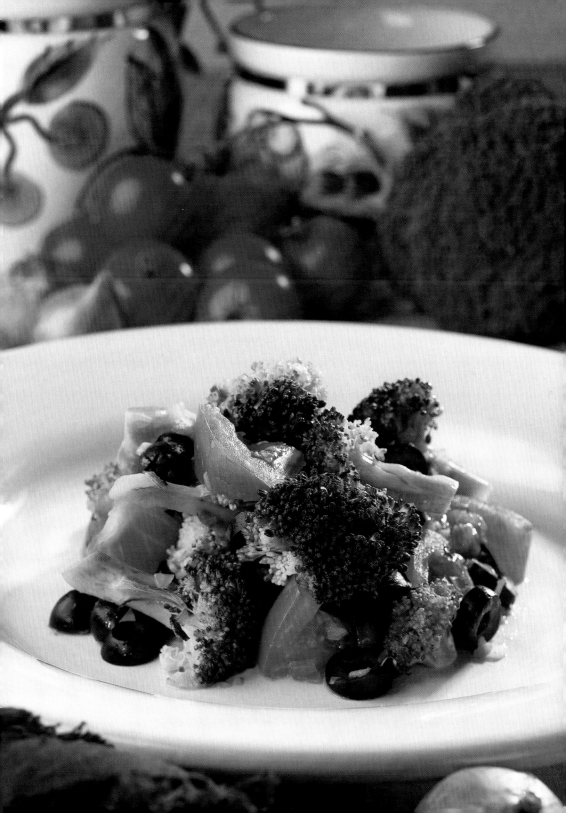

Artichoke Herb Dip

This delicious dip is best made with fresh artichokes, but you can also use a medium-size jar (430 g) of artichokes in water.

4 artichokes

Juice of a lemon

2 tbsp flax oil

4 cloves garlic, minced

1 shallot, minced

½ cup (125 ml) kefir

1½ tsp Dijon mustard

1 tbsp sunflower oil

fresh chopped herbs - basil, dill and/or tarragon, thyme

1½ tsp capers

Tamari soy sauce, to taste

Sea salt, to taste

Wash the artichokes, remove the stems and tips with scissors and brush lemon juice on the cut edges. Steam the artichokes over boiling water for 20 minutes or until tender. Artichokes are cooked when you can easily pull out an inner leaf.

Remove leaves and bottom part of artichokes, leaving only the hearts. Put hearts in blender with all remaining ingredients. Blend on slow speed to start and then on high speed until smooth.

Serves 2

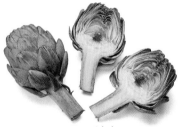

artichoke

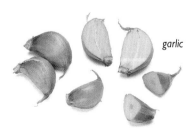

garlic

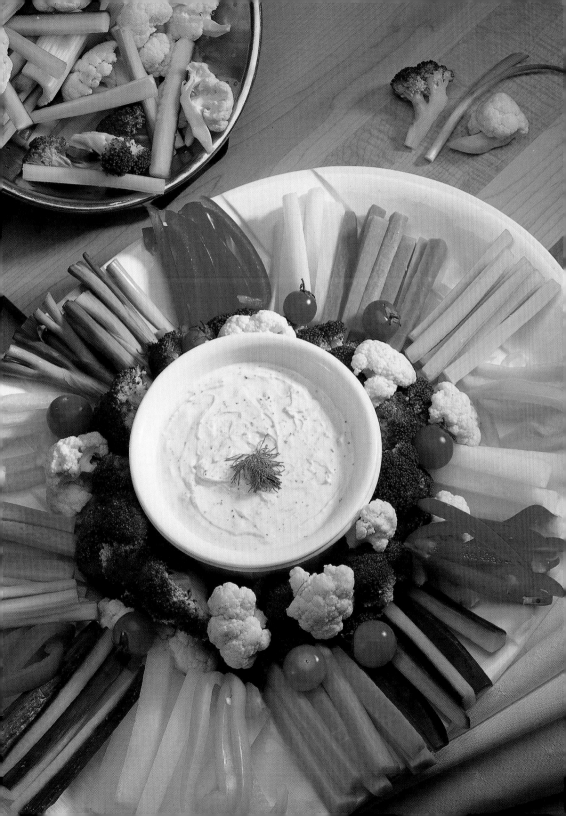

Cashew Cheese Spread

This spread is delicious on top of whole-grain crackers, baked potatoes or steamed vegetables. The agar agar gives a gelatin-like consistency.

1½ **tsp** (10 g)
  agar agar powder

3 tbsp cold water

1½ **cups** (600 g)
  raw cashews

½ **cup** (200 g)
  sunflower seeds

**2 tbsp nutritional yeast
  (optional)**

1 tsp sea salt

**1 tbsp freshly squeezed
  lemon juice**

3 tbsp finely grated carrot

**1 tbsp flax seed or
  sunflower seed oil**

In a small saucepan stir the agar agar into cold water and soften it over very low heat. Mix all the ingredients in the blender, one half at a time to achieve an even texture. Blend until creamy. Thoroughly mix the two batches together and pour into a mold or bowl. Chill in the refrigerator.

Serves 3-4

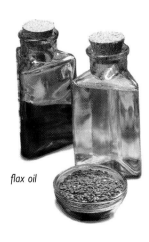

flax oil

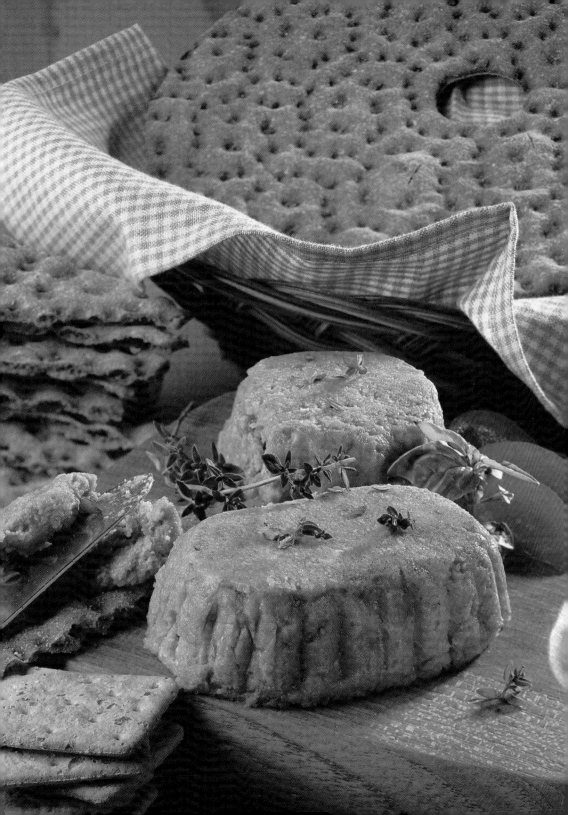

Sunflower Seed and Vegetable Paté

This perfect party food can also be served with steamed vegetables, baked potatoes or yams for a light family meal.

1½ cups (600 g) **sunflower seeds, freshly ground**

¾ **cup** (200 g) **whole-wheat flour**

¾ **cup** (200 g) **nutritional yeast**

1 **tbsp each fresh thyme and basil, finely chopped**

1 **tsp fresh sage, finely chopped**

1 **tsp sea salt**

2 **cups** (400 g) **potato, freshly grated**

½ **cup** (125 ml) **extra-virgin olive oil**

2 **cups** (500 ml) **warm water**

2 **cups** (300 g) **chopped leeks or mild onions**

Juice of 2 medium-size lemons

Preheat the oven to 350°F (190°C).

Thoroughly mix the seeds, flour, yeast, herbs and salt in a large bowl. Add the potato and oil, mix again, then stir in water, leeks and lemon juice. Spread the paté mixture into an ungreased 8" x 8" (20 cm x 20 cm) pan and bake in the oven for 1 hour.

Serves 10

Variation:

A garlic cream sauce makes this a really special dish to serve guests.

1 **cup** (250 ml) **cream or raw milk**

1 **tbsp whole-wheat flour**

1 **or more garlic cloves, grated**

In a saucepan, heat the cream with the garlic. Moisten the flour to a paste with a little water and slowly add to the cream. Cook until just thickened.

To prevent oxidation, be sure to grate the potatoes just before mixing into the leeks and lemon juice.

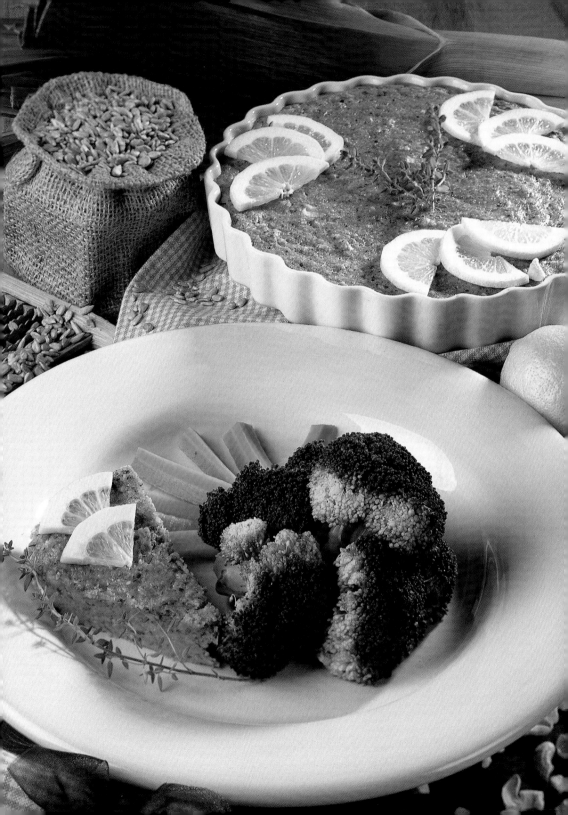

Rhody's Health Combo

This tasty liver-cleansing vegetable juice combines antioxidant-rich root vegetables and greens.

3 medium-size carrots

1 medium-size beet root

3 or 4 dandelion leaves

Small piece of ginger

1 or 2 large celery stalks

Juice all ingredients according to the directions for your juicing machine. Serve immediately.

Serves 1

Variation
Add a half cup of kefir to your fresh juice.

> If you're like me and hate to throw out any food, you can make a broth using the vegetable pulp. Add chopped onions, a few onion skins and a chopped potato to the pulp and simmer in 4 or 5 cups of distilled or purified water for a half hour. Throw away the pulp and keep the stock for soup or for a mineral drink, adding a heaping teaspoonful of powdered greens.

Aunt Rhody's Seedy Soup and Salad Topping

I've been making this nut and seed topping for years. I like to sprinkle it on salads, soup and vegetables. The ingredients listed are all equal parts or according to your taste. Use a coffee grinder or spice mill to grind the seeds.

**Nutritional yeast,
  powdered or flaked**

Psyllium husks, powdered

Chia seeds, freshly ground

Flax seeds, freshly ground

**Sunflower seeds,
  freshly ground**

**Sesame seeds, lightly
  toasted in an iron pan**

**Fennel seeds,
  freshly ground**

In a bowl, mix together all ingredients. Put this topping on your table and sprinkle on just about everything.

Variation
Mix this topping with a little kefir and flax seed oil and use it as a vegetable dip or a bread spread.

Lecithin granules

Dulse flakes

Dash of cayenne pepper, or to taste

Garlic salt (optional)

> Seeds taste best when they're freshly ground, so don't make too large a quantity at once. You should store this topping in a dark glass jar in the freezer to prevent the fatty acids in the flax seeds from going rancid.

references

Cabot, Sandra.
The Healthy Liver & Bowel Book
Australia: WHAS, 1999.

Cabot, Sandra.
The Liver Cleansing Diet
Scottsdale, AZ: S.C.B. International, 1996.

Christopher, John R.
School of Natural Healing
Provo, Ut: BiWorld Publishers, Inc., 1976

Kloss, Jethro
Back to Eden
California: Loma Linden, 1988

Gursche, Siegfried
Juicing for the Health of It!
Vancouver, BC: Alive Publishing Group Inc., 2000

sources

for organic extra virgin coconut oil, household health equipment, juicers, sprouters, blenders, and more:
Alpha Health Products
7434 Fraser Park Dr.
Burnaby, BC V5J 5B9 Canada
Tel: 800-663-2212
www.alphahealth.ca

For Milk Thistle Plus, Liver Cleanse Kit, Dandelion Tea & other liver cleansing support products, digestive aids, probiotics, unrefined organic oils:
Flora Manufacturing & Distributing Ltd.
7400 Fraser Park Drive
Burnaby, BC VJ 5B9 Canada
604-436-6000
888-436-6697 (product information)
www.florahealth.com

for Bali's Sun organic extra virgin coconut oil:
Jimar Enterprises Ltd.
PB/CP 45023, Laval, QC Canada
Tel: 888-969-1874
coco@balissun.com
www.balissun.com

for water filters & precision water distiller:
Polar Bear Health Equipment
9342-118th Avenue
Edmonton, AB T5G 0N4
800-661-9954 or 780-477-1328
www.polarbearhealth.com

for unrefined organic oils:
Rapunzel Pure Organics Inc
2424 State Route 203
Valatie, NY 12184 USA
800-207-2814 or 518-392-86-20
info@rapunzel.com
www.rapunzel.com

First published in 2000 by
alive books
7432 Fraser Park Drive
Burnaby BC V5J 5B9
(604) 435-1919
1-800-661-0303

© 2000 by **alive** books
Eighth Printing – January 2005

Book Design:
    Paul Chau
Artwork:
    Terence Yeung
    Raymond Cheung
    Liza Novecoski
Food Styling:
    Fred Edrissi
Photography:
    Edmond Fong
    (food photography)
    Siegfried Gursche
Photo Editing:
    Sabine Edrissi-Bredenbrock
Editing:
    Sandra Tonn
    Julie Cheng

Canadian Cataloguing in Publication Data

Lake, Rhody
    Liver Cleansing Handbook

(**alive** natural health guides, 4
ISSN 1490-6503)
ISBN 1-55312-004-3

Printed in Canada

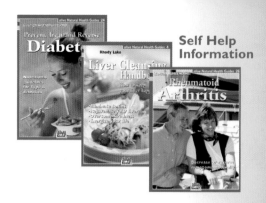
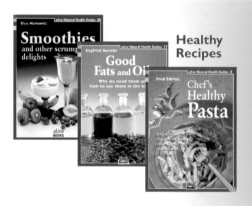
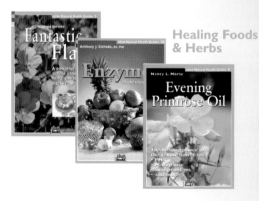
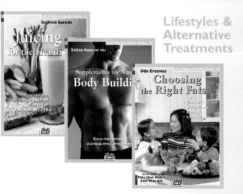